THE BOOK OF
NEUROPOETRY

DR. STEPHEN PETERS

THE BOOK OF NEUROPOETRY

DR. STEPHEN PETERS

WASTELAND PRESS
www.wastelandpress.net

Wasteland Press

www.wastelandpress.net
Shelbyville, KY USA

The Book of Neuropoetry
by Dr. Stephen Peters

First Printing – June 2025
Paperback ISBN: 978-1-68111-603-7
Hardback ISBN: 978-1-68111-604-4
LCCN: to be determined
Back Cover Photograph by Michelle Snook

Printed in the U.S.A.

0 1 2 3

For Kip and Michelle

"To create or perceive beauty is to change the brain—each line drawn becomes a thread in the fabric of perception, leaving a trace on the quiet witness."

—Dr. Stephen Peters

AUTHOR'S FOREWORD

A shared language of horses, nervous systems, science, and soul. Where poetry becomes a portal, and the signal beneath words is heard.

This is not a book I wrote alone. These words—these poems, reflections, and insights—arose from something far more vast than I. They came quietly, often without warning. Some arrived on long walks through the canyons and high country of Colorado, Kip trotting beside me. Others drifted in while I lay half-asleep in the soft warmth of an afternoon nap. Still others surfaced in the hush of meditation, or in the instant clarity that follows a question asked not to the world, but to the Universe itself. This book was co-authored by that very presence—call it the Universe, the field, the collective unconscious, or simply the deep intelligence of nature. I do not claim ownership of many of these words. They passed through me, not from me. I am their vessel, not their architect.

In these pages, horses speak in the language of neuroscience. The soul is seen through the lens of the synapse. Art and biology, perception and presence, mystery and method—all take their turn in the saddle. This is not merely a book about the nervous system. It is a living record of what can happen when science bows to wonder, and when a mind quiets long enough to listen.

What Is Neuropoetry? Why This Book Now?

What if a poem could do more than move you?
What if it could modulate your nervous system—
invite your breath to slow,
your attention to deepen,
your brain to rewire?

This is the promise of neuropoetry.

I have spent my career inside the folds and firings of the brain—human and equine. As a neuroscientist and clinician, I have dissected brains, studied neurotransmitters, and charted neural circuits. But in recent years, something unexpected began to emerge: poetry. Not as a departure from science, but as its natural complement.

Poetry, it turns out, speaks the brain's native language: rhythm, imagery, pattern, and emotional salience. These are not embellishments. They are *entrances*—gateways into deeper learning and healing. A well-tuned line of verse can downshift arousal, awaken interoception, and even stimulate the very plasticity that allows change to occur.

In an age of disconnection—where attention is fractured, stress is chronic, and language often serves more to divide than to heal—I offer this book as a bridge. Between science and soul. Between fact and feeling. Between what we *know* about the brain and what we can *feel* from it.

Several poems in this collection are followed by a brief clinical postscript. Think of it as a glimpse behind the curtain—a translation of poetry back into biology. These reflections are not meant to explain the poems, but to ground them. To reveal the anatomy beneath the metaphor, the neurochemistry inside the moment.

You'll find horses here. And humans. And sometimes both at once. You'll find fear and awe, memory and learning, sleep and arousal, stillness and signal. You may even find yourself reflected—in a synapse, in a trail, in a breath.

This is not just a book about the nervous system. It is written *with* the nervous system in mind. And perhaps, if we've done our work well, it will speak not only to your intellect, but to the felt intelligence of your senses.

Welcome to the *The Book of Neuropoetry.*

Dr. Stephen Peters
Mancos, Colorado
2025

INTRODUCTORY NOTE

This is not a book with a table of contents.

There are no chapters or categories. No prescribed order. That's intentional.

The brain doesn't work like a list—it shifts between systems, responds to the environment, and makes meaning through patterns and experience. This book mirrors that.

Each poem stands on its own.
Some explore stress and regulation. Others focus on connection, memory, perception, or the biology of emotion. The science is real, but the poems are meant to be experienced, not analyzed.

You don't need to read it from beginning to end.
Open to a page. Follow your interest. Come back later. What resonates today may feel different tomorrow.

This is a book to support awareness, reflection, and change.
It offers a new way of seeing the nervous system—through language that moves, quiets, and connects.

You're invited to explore, not just read.
And in doing so, to participate in something we're all capable of: ongoing neural change and co-evolution.

Shared Current

On Co-Creation and Neural Synchrony

Between two beings,
a filament forms—
not seen,
but sensed—
a field shaped
by motion,
by timing,
by trust.

You shift your weight,
they feel it.
They blink,
you respond.
This is how dialogue begins—
through presence
before pressure,
through rhythm
before reason.

Inside both bodies,
the chemistry listens.
Oxytocin steadies the field,
dopamine pulses with anticipation,
acetylcholine sharpens the moment.

You are not leading—
you are joining.
Not commanding—
but composing,

a duet of nervous systems
writing the present together.

Each breath you take
can shape their state.
Each signal you send
is both intention
and invitation.

Synchrony is not technique.
It is truth
felt across skin,
shared in silence,
co-authored
in the space between.

Clinical Postscript

This poem portrays synchrony as a co-authored experience—a moment-by-moment neural dialogue between horse and human. From a neuroscience perspective, such interactions are underpinned by dynamic exchanges between two social nervous systems. Communication in this context is more than behavioral; it is neurochemical, autonomic, and somatic.

When a human approaches with calm intention, oxytocin may rise in both species, promoting a sense of safety and social receptivity. Acetylcholine contributes to focused, non-reactive attention, enabling both beings to stay present without tipping into hyperarousal. Dopamine enhances the motivational salience of interaction, preparing both partners to learn from and anticipate meaningful patterns. Norepinephrine modulates alertness, attuning each brain to subtle shifts in the other's signals.

This co-regulatory process allows mutual adjustment in posture, breath, muscle tone, and affect. Synchrony doesn't arise from controlling the other—it emerges when each system is both clear and responsive. To participate in this shared current is to be emotionally regulated, somatically aware, and neurobiologically honest.

What looks like seamless partnership from the outside is, in truth, the visible surface of deeply layered neural resonance.

To Be Seen by a Horse

on perception, projection, and the silent science between species

The horse does not speak—
but perceives
through skin, through sinew,
through the fine-tuned receptors
of eye, ear, and vibrissae.

She reads the world
in scent and shadow,
in pressure and posture,
in the shape of silence
before a sound is made.

She sees your posture
before your words,
feels the charge
before the command.

A flicker of your pupil,
a shift in your spine—
these are volumes to her,
even when you
don't realize
you are being read aloud.

She hears tension
not in your voice,
but in the cadence
of your silence.

To you, she is stubborn,
reactive, distracted—
but what if she is
interpreting you
with a nervous system
older and wiser
than your language?

What if the refusal
is not disobedience,
but discernment—
a body declining to mirror
your dysregulation?

You gaze at her
with narrowed cognition,
seeking signs that match
your story.
But she—
she sees all of you.
Even the parts
you hide from yourself.

The misstep,
the stillness,
the wide-eyed turn—
these are her replies.

Not resistance,
but response.
Not misbehavior,
but misunderstood perception.

She is not here
to be shaped by your agenda—
but to reveal
what it's like
to be seen
by a sensory system
that doesn't lie.

Clinical Postscript

A horse's sensory world is fundamentally different from ours—panoramic vision, acute motion detection, vibrissae tuned for close tactile input, and an auditory range adapted for survival. Their nervous system is designed to process nuance long before overt behavior emerges.

When horses react, they are often responding to stimuli we've failed to notice—our tone, micro-movements, inner states. This poem challenges anthropocentric interpretations and invites us to recognize that horses are not faulty mirrors—they are precise instruments. To understand them, we must first recalibrate ourselves.

The Brain Chooses Safety

He doesn't care who's boss.
Not in the way we think.

In the horse's brain,
hierarchy is not a ladder—
it's a landscape of signals.
Every step, every touch
asks the same question:
Am I safe here?

The limbic system doesn't parse intention,
only experience.
Your pressure may feel like a predator.
Your silence, a snare.

He doesn't test you.
He reads you.
Faster than thought.
Before your words arrive,
his nervous system already knows.

You may get obedience
through tension,
but learning lives
in the quiet between threats—
where dopamine drips,
where the hippocampus listens.

Real leadership isn't taken.
It's offered—
through clarity,
consistency,
and co-regulation.

Ask not if he respects you,
but if his breath is steady near you.
That is the only measure
his brain believes.

Clinical Postscript

Dominance-based approaches ignore the equine brain's core imperative: safety. *The amygdala flags threat milliseconds before cognition. When fear is present, the hippocampus may encode vivid, emotionally charged memories—but not necessarily in ways that support adaptive learning. In fact, under high stress, the brain may bypass the basal ganglia's habit systems, reverting to reflex and reactivity rather than thoughtful response.*

In contrast, calm states allow acetylcholine to support attention, dopamine to foster motivation, and oxytocin to nurture social trust. True leadership emerges not from command, but from co-regulation—creating the neurological conditions where learning can occur, and where connection is not a strategy, but a state.

The Listening Brain

We live in a world where sound never stops.
Yet the art of listening remains profoundly rare.
The horse—a creature of prey—
listens not just with its ears,
but with its nervous system.
It listens for safety, for subtlety, for sincerity.
And what about us?
The human brain—
complex, pattern-seeking, ever-adaptive—
filters signal from noise with astonishing precision.
Attention, guided by acetylcholine, sharpens our focus.
Emotion, balanced by serotonin, steadies our lens.
Motivation, driven by dopamine, fuels our curiosity.
These are not abstractions.
They are the neurochemical symphony behind every moment of understanding.
And in the quiet space between words—
that is where true connection begins.
Not with dominance. Not with force.
But with presence. With patience. With trust.
In the end, the brain learns best—
not under threat,
but through clarity.
And yet—
under the right conditions,
with safety, trust, and repetition,
both horses and humans
can learn to find coherence,
even in the midst of chaos.

Thinking Like a Neurologist

for those who seek truth inside the signal

Don't rush to name the shadow—
watch how it moves.
Truth lives not in labels,
but in the rhythm of pattern.

Begin not with answers,
but with questions shaped like tuning forks:
Where does the signal start?
What path does it follow?

The horse stumbles—
not always from weakness,
but perhaps from a disconnection,
or a memory misfired
along circuits worn by stress.

A twitch is not always a tic.
A silence is not always peace.
A change in behavior
may be a whispered cry from the brainstem,
not a battle of wills.

Confirmation is seductive.
It nods quickly—
too quickly.
But the neurologist waits.
Watches.
Returns to first principles.

Under the skin,
in the long corridors of the cord,
there is always a story.
But not always the one you expect.

So don't fall in love
with your first theory.
Marry observation.
Date doubt.
And walk the nervous system
as if it were a forest
that will not reveal its truths
until you've walked it twice—
once with knowledge,
and once with the neutrality
of a mind trained to observe before it names.

Clinical Postscript

This poem reflects the clinical mindset of a neurologist: resisting premature conclusions, tolerating ambiguity, and staying attuned to patterns over isolated symptoms.

In both human and equine neurology, diagnostic clarity often emerges not from a single finding, but from how *signs relate over time, space, and function.*

Critical thinking in this field is not a trait—it's a practice: observing before naming, questioning before confirming, and understanding that the nervous system rarely lies, but often speaks in code.

Three Quiet Moments

A neuropoetic trilogy of presence

When the Horse Stood Still

The field was empty
except for the horse—
head low, tail soft as grass,
one hoof resting
like a thought half-formed.

I stood by the fence,
the day still loud in my chest,
but she—
did nothing.

No performance.
No explanation.
Only the quiet rhythm
of a body at peace
with the wind.

Something in me
let go without ceremony.
I felt it—
not in words,
but in how time stopped
counting.

She did not move.
And slowly,
I began to unfold

into the space
she had already found.

The Wild Keeps Time

No one was speaking.
Not the wind
through the narrow grass,
not the hawk
spiraling out of sight.

I walked without aim,
just the soft rhythm
of boots on earth—
and somewhere behind me,
the dog
stitching silence with joy.

A horse lifted her head
from grazing,
watched for a moment,
then returned to what mattered.

The sun moved
without asking
if I was ready.
The sky changed
without apology.

And I—
nervous system unwinding—
began to feel
less like a visitor.

The air cooled
as if breath itself
were shared
among all things.

And in that still hour,
I knew:
the wild keeps time
in its own way—
not by clocks,
but by what the body
remembers
when the mind
finally stops interrupting.

Kip at the Edge of the Meadow

(for the one who lives to please)

She runs ahead,
then arcs back—
never straying far,
as if my breath
were a tether.

Nose low,
ears tuned to the world,
she moves
with a kind of listening
only devotion understands.

Every glance she gives
asks the same question—
Am I with you?
And my smallest nod
becomes her whole reward.

She waits for it—
the soft yes in my voice,
the quiet click
of things being right again.

When I say her name,
she comes
like a promise kept—
swift and bright,
her whole body answering.

She doesn't just follow—
she aligns.
The space between us
fills with something
warm and true.

And when she leans
her black-and-white frame
against my leg,
I feel a slowing inside—
as if my own heart,
hearing hers,
decided to stay awhile
and rest.

Clinical Postscript

In these moments—when a horse stands still, when a dog returns to your side, when the wild carries you without demand—you are not merely witnessing peace; you are participating in it. These poems speak in the quiet language of a nervous system at ease—of oxytocin and safety, of attunement without speech, of regulation found not through control, but through connection. This is where the brain softens. This is where rewiring begins. Not in effort, but in presence.

The Shape of Awe

(on neuroaesthetics and the perception of beauty)

Some things feel right
before we can explain why—
the curve of a shell,
a chord resolving,
sunlight slanting through late-afternoon air.

It isn't magic.
It's pattern.
The brain searches for order,
and rewards its discovery.

Symmetry, proportion, contrast—
these aren't just aesthetic choices.
They're signals.
Hints of safety,
coherence,
fitness.

The orbitofrontal cortex assigns value.
The visual cortex sharpens its focus.
Dopamine follows form.

Even the right shade of yellow—
like Van Gogh's sunflowers—
can settle something inside us
we didn't know was restless.

What we call beauty
might be the nervous system

recognizing efficiency.
A cue that says:
This fits. You can stop searching.

And in that moment,
perception becomes pleasure.
Not escape—
but understanding.

Clinical Postscript

Neuroaesthetics explores why certain stimuli—visual, auditory, or tactile—resonate deeply within the brain. Research shows that symmetry, proportion, contrast, *and* predictable patterns *often activate the orbitofrontal cortex, a region involved in evaluating reward and emotional valence. The fusiform gyrus is engaged in the recognition of faces and familiar forms, and dopaminergic pathways are activated when a stimulus is perceived as pleasing or meaningful.*

These responses are not arbitrary. From an evolutionary standpoint, the ability to detect harmony and coherence in our environment may have conferred survival advantages—identifying health in a mate, safety in a landscape, or intention in movement.

Beauty, then, is not merely decorative. It is informational. It signals fit, fluency, and sometimes even emotional truth. Whether it's a lead change in a horse, the precise interval in music, or the balanced composition of a painting, the experience of beauty is often the brain's way of saying: This makes sense.

In this way, awe is not an escape from the world, but a deep alignment with it.

Beautiful When It Shouldn't Be

(on the neuroaesthetics of surprise)

You weren't expecting it—
the note that doesn't resolve,
the painting that breaks the rules,
the wild turn in a familiar trail.

It catches you,
not with comfort,
but with something stranger—
attention sharpened,
breath held.

The brain registers error.
And then—
re-evaluates.

Novelty floods the salience network.
The anterior cingulate leans in.
This doesn't match the model.
But it matters.

When what's unfamiliar
reveals a deeper order,
the reward is doubled.

Now beauty isn't recognition.
It's discovery.
It's the moment when the nervous system says:
I didn't expect that...
but I'm glad I saw it.

A horse moving like water
after years of stiffness.
A face once overlooked
suddenly full of light.

This is beauty
not because it repeats,
but because it rewrites.

Clinical Postscript

Beauty is not always born of symmetry or familiarity. Sometimes, the most profound aesthetic experiences arise from surprise—when the brain encounters a stimulus that violates its predictions yet reveals meaning.

This is where the salience network—particularly the anterior cingulate cortex and insula—comes into play. These regions monitor for novelty, uncertainty, and relevance. When something unexpected carries emotional or sensory weight, attention locks in. The brain shifts from default mode into active processing.

If the unexpected input turns out to be coherent or valuable—such as an unconventional musical phrase, an asymmetrical face with striking character, or a moment of grace in a being once overlooked—dopaminergic reward systems are activated. This coupling of prediction error with positive valuation creates a heightened sense of awe or aesthetic pleasure.

Neuroaesthetics tells us that beauty isn't just about what fits the mold. It can also arise from what breaks it—when the nervous system is surprised, and that surprise turns into insight.

This is beauty as revelation.

Effortless Knowing

There comes a moment
when you no longer reach for it—
it reaches through you.

The act,
once carved
by prefrontal strain,
now glides
along myelinated tracks
laid down by devotion.

The basal ganglia hums
like a trusted engine,
its circuits silent
but sure.

What began with sweat and error,
fired and fired again,
now rests in synaptic certainty—
LTP etched
each pathway
into permanence.

What once took thought
now takes form.
It flows
like water knows the riverbed.

You do not think
to breathe,

or blink,
or balance.
So too
this motion—
this feel,
this timing—
becomes embedded.

No need for language.
No room for doubt.
The self is absent,
and so is fear.

I saw it once
before I moved—
not with my eyes,
but with intention's shadow.

And then
I vanished,
replaced
by the rhythm
of rightness.

Clinical Postscript

This poem reflects the neural mechanics of embodied expertise. With practice, repeated synaptic activity triggers long-term potentiation (LTP)—a mechanism of learning in which neural connections are strengthened and stabilized. Myelination of frequently used axons increases conduction velocity, allowing actions to flow with less conscious oversight. As procedural memory consolidates, control shifts from the prefrontal cortex to the basal ganglia, enabling automaticity. Visualization alone can reinforce motor networks, priming execution. During flow states, transient hypofrontality quiets self-referential processing while acetylcholine and dopamine modulate attention and reward. In this space, skill becomes seamless, and awareness becomes embodiment.

The Brain That Walks Toward Light

(on neuroplasticity and lived experience)

The brain is not fixed.
It listens.
It shapes itself
by what we do,
where we go,
and how we feel when we get there.

Dendrites reach
toward repeated signals.
Axons trace
the rhythms of our days.
Experience becomes structure—
not metaphorically,
but physically.

New paths form
in movement,
in relationship,
in attention given without urgency.

Safety allows branching.
Curiosity strengthens it.
What fires together,
wires together—
a living architecture
of becoming.

The brain does not ask,
Is this right?
It asks,
Is this real, and will it be happening again?

And so,
with each moment of presence,
a new pattern takes shape.
This is not repair.
This is growth
by design.

Clinical Postscript

Neuroplasticity is the brain's capacity to shape itself through experience. From moment to moment, neural circuits are strengthened, pruned, or newly formed in response to what we do, sense, feel, and imagine.

Plasticity is not reserved for moments of change—it is the mechanism of change. With each repetition, the brain refines its predictions. With each novel encounter, it expands its capacity. Dendrites branch, synapses form, myelin wraps new highways of communication. Glial cells support this remodeling—nourishing, regulating, and maintaining neural health.

In environments rich with safety, exploration, and meaningful engagement, plasticity flourishes. The brain isn't passively recording the world—it is actively building it, encoding relationships, movements, ideas, and sensations into the architecture of the self.

Neuroplasticity is how we become who we are. It is the process of living translated into structure. And it reminds us that with every experience, we are never truly finished—we are in formation.

Introduction to Constructed Realities

We do not passively perceive the world—we build it.
Moment by moment, our brains are engaged in a quiet, continuous act of construction. What we feel, see, and understand is filtered through past experience, bodily sensation, and predicted meaning. This is true not only for humans, but for horses as well.

Modern neuroscience reveals that emotion is not simply a reaction—it is an interpretation. The brain anticipates what is likely to happen next, shaping perception and behavior in service of survival. This predictive processing occurs beneath conscious awareness, relying heavily on interoception (the sense of the internal body), context, and repetition.

For the horse—whose life is so often dictated by human environments—this understanding is vital. The stall, the rope, the raised voice—none exist in isolation. They are interpreted through the lens of memory and expectation, just as we interpret our world through stories built upon layers of learned meaning.

The following two poems explore this concept of constructed reality—first through the lens of human consciousness, then through the lived neurobiology of the horse. Together, they ask us to reconsider how we experience the world, and how we shape the world for others—especially those without a voice to explain what they feel.

Constructed Realities

(inspired by the spirit of existential neurobiology)

You awaken inside a framework
you never consciously chose—
a place, a role, a rhythm
built not by intention,
but by prediction.

Maps unfold beneath you
written in the language
of past experience.
You travel them as if by choice,
but the routes were drawn
before awareness caught up.

Your hands steer
through memories shaped as highways,
your body responding
to signals beneath language—
glimpses of purpose,
flashes of confusion.

And you ask,
not with logic, but with ache:
How did I arrive at this version of myself?

Beneath that question,
a deeper current flows—
affective tides
not seen,
but felt.

Emotion begins as sensation—
temperature, tension, breath—
and only later becomes
a story.

You float on a sea
of neural forecasting—
the brain, always guessing,
trying to make the world
fit what it already believes.

Repetition feels like safety,
even when it's not.
Familiarity—
a chemical balm
for an uncertain world.

Yet under all certainties
there is motion.
Even stillness moves.
The brain,
an organ of becoming,
never rests—
constructing, refining,
explaining the action
only after it's done.

Meaning isn't discovered—
it's manufactured
in the silent chambers
of cortical narration.

You think you're remembering.
You're actually reassembling.
You think you're perceiving.
You're actually predicting.

In the moment of reckoning,
you may pause—
not to find the truth,
but to feel the hum
of constructed reality
and recognize
that it is not fixed.
It never was.

The self is water-shaped—
a temporary sculpture
of neurons and need,
held together
by what you expect to feel.

Neuroconstruct: The Horse Between Worlds

A companion to "Constructed Realities"

The horse does not live
in some mythic now—
untouched by memory,
free from the past.

No.
He lives in a body
that remembers.

Every hoof-fall
echoes through layers
of prediction—
tactile, vestibular, visceral—
each step guided by
what has come before.

He does not *see* a rope—
he feels the shadow
of what ropes have meant.
He does not *hear* your voice—
he measures its tone
against a thousand tones
that preceded it.

His brain is not waiting
to be triggered.
It is already forecasting—

matching sight with consequence,
touch with tale,
gesture with gut.

In every moment,
his nervous system whispers:
Have I felt this before?
What did it mean?
What did I do?

He lives in *constructed immediacy*—
not just reacting,
but assembling the present
through the filter of experience.

That pause before he moves?
Not stubbornness—
but simulation.
A surge of interoception
and autonomic signals
cross-checking prediction
with unfolding now.

His vigilance
is not just instinct.
It is a rehearsal
of remembered uncertainty.

His stillness
is not absence.
It is processing.

And trust—
when it arrives—
is not gifted.

It is grown
through enough consistency
to rewire what the past
once warned.

For the horse,
safety is not a stall.
It is a pattern of freedom—
a field with room to notice,
to choose,
to breathe.

Emotion is not a flare.
It is a forecast,
shaped by context,
calm,
and consistency.

And the human—
to be meaningful—
must enter not just the pasture,
but the process—
respecting the brain
beneath the mane.

The Hallucination We Agree to Call Real

on perception, prediction, and the theater of the mind

You do not see the world as it is—
you see it as you've been.
Each moment a mosaic
stitched from whispers deep within.

Light arrives in scattered rays,
but you don't perceive the light—
you see what memory allows,
what matches inner night.

The scent of rain on asphalt heat
is not the smell alone,
but childhood storms and summers lost,
a feeling you've outgrown.

Your ears take in a crowded room,
but filter every voice
through neural weights of relevance—
you do not hear, you *make* a choice.

The world arrives in static bursts,
ambiguous and blurred—
your brain, the grand interpreter,
assigns it shape and word.

It builds with prior scaffolding,
with expectation's thread—

projecting futures into now,
constructing what's ahead.

This isn't trick or flaw or sin—
it's how we've learned to be:
to render noise intelligible,
to simulate and see.

But take heart in this illusion,
this curated display:
your brain can recompose the scene
and paint a different day.

For you are not a fixed design—
your map is made, then redrawn.
You are the artist of your sight,
the dreamer before the dawn.

And if the world appears too stark,
too cruel, too sharp, too small—
remember: this hallucination
was never fixed at all.

Clinical Postscript

On Perception and Predictive Brain Function

Modern neuroscience increasingly shows that perception is not a passive recording of reality but an active, brain-based construction. In every moment, your brain is bombarded with ambiguous, noisy data from the senses. To make sense of this influx, it relies on internal models—shaped by past experiences, context, and learned expectations—to generate predictions about what's most likely happening out there in the world.

This process—known as predictive processing or active inference—means we don't perceive the world directly. Instead, we experience a "best guess" shaped by prior experience and constantly updated through sensory input. As Anil Seth puts it, perception is a controlled hallucination: a reality sculpted from the inside out.

Becoming Through the Senses

You bite the fruit.
Not just to feed,
but to remember ripeness,
and teach your brain
what sweetness feels like.

You walk beneath pines,
each footfall a conversation
with gravity and earth —
the rhythm of movement
rehearsing presence.

Warm water touches your skin,
and your nervous system listens —
not for language,
but for safety,
for permission to soften.

You reach for a friend,
not just for words,
but for the echo of being seen —
because to be held
is to become.

These are not moments.
They are instructions.
And the brain —
forever listening —
rewires accordingly.

Clinical Postscript

The human brain constructs experience by predicting and interpreting sensory input through the lens of prior learning. This continuous loop — experience shaping perception, perception shaping future experience — lies at the heart of neuroplasticity.

Each sensory moment becomes an opportunity for rewiring. When one "bites into ripe fruit," it is not just a metabolic act but an emotional encoding. The sweetness — mediated in part by dopaminergic pathways — teaches the brain what is safe, rewarding, and life-enhancing. It helps form templates of joy and nourishment that inform future predictions and behaviors.

To "walk beneath trees" is more than locomotion; it is "rehearsing presence". Rhythmic, embodied movement activates networks in the cerebellum and basal ganglia that regulate attention, motor coordination, and internal timing. Such movement-based rituals reinforce the neural circuits that support grounded awareness — a practice of returning to now.

To seek "the echo of being seen" is to engage in one of the most powerful experiences the nervous system knows: attuned social connection. Through relational resonance — via the mirror neuron system, anterior cingulate, and medial prefrontal cortex — the brain encodes the experience of being understood, valued, and safe. This leaves an imprint that shapes identity and emotional regulation over time.

These moments — whether sensory or relational — are not passive. They are active sculptors of the brain. And because thought, behavior, and environmental exposure can influence gene expression through epigenetic mechanisms, the lifestyle one chooses becomes a form of intentional evolution. This is how we build a meaningful, healthy, and adaptive life — not just from what we do, but from how deeply we feel it.

An Intimate Afternoon

after the pulse, before the pastry

Slowly—
in the hush between noon and sigh,
when the ceiling fan breathes lullabies
and time itself forgets to press,
they meet in tangled, fragrant flesh.

Calcium floods the waiting gate,
a voltage shift, a change in state.
Sodium rushes down the line—
an axon spark, a spine-to-spine.

Her skin, a page of heat and print,
reads fingertip like Braille in glint.
Receptors sing in silent throng,
each touch a phosphene, bright and long.

Glutamate's wild scatter spills,
dopamine climbs pleasure's hills.
Oxytocin braids their breath—
each exhale softens fear of death.

He whispers into folds of hair,
where scent and sweat compose a prayer.
Noradrenaline gives way to grace,
as parasympathy takes its place.

No climax shouts—no need for flight,
but deep entrainment, dappled light.
Even the sheets seem to align
with rhythms buried deep in time.

Then stillness. Then
the fork dips low
into a peach too ripe to hold.
Its nectar clings to teeth and tongue,
a sun-warmed syrup gently sung.

Crumbs of croissant fall like snow
upon her collarbone below.
He wipes them with a lover's care,
a laugh, a kiss, a grateful stare.

Bitterness from coffee's rim
dances with sugar's playful hymn.
The quiet hum of resting brain
begins to dream its dream again—

Of bodies as electric land,
of language shaped by breath, not hand.
Of how two nervous systems find
a moment's peace in shared design.

And though this hour cannot stay,
its memory will branch and play—
encoded deep, not stored above,
a neuron's echo made from love.

Clinical Postscript

Companion Note: The Neurobiology of Intimate Memory

This poem traces not only the sensual experience of two lovers but the layered choreography of their nervous systems in union. Touch, scent, rhythm, and reciprocity become electrical and chemical dialogues—each sensation sparking cascades of activity from peripheral receptors to cortical association networks.

During physical intimacy, a symphony of neurotransmitters is released. Dopamine fuels pleasure and motivation, reinforcing the behaviors that brought about connection. Oxytocin, often called the bonding hormone, deepens trust and emotional safety, enhancing the feeling of unity. Glutamate, the brain's primary excitatory neurotransmitter, ensures that sensory signals are amplified and etched into memory. And as the sympathetic arousal begins to ebb, the parasympathetic nervous system—governor of rest, digestion, and restoration—reclaims the body, allowing for relaxation, nourishment, and contentment.

Post-coital states are not just biochemical wind-downs—they're windows into neural consolidation. Experiences like the sweetness of fruit, the softness of sheets, and the quiet of afternoon light become anchored into episodic memory through hippocampal-cortical replay—a brain-wide integration process during calm, reflective states. These "small" moments, often overlooked, are the very ones that shape intimacy, identity, and the felt sense of being known.

In this poem, love is not metaphor alone—it is transmission, reception, entrainment, and co-regulation. Two nervous systems, briefly but profoundly, find coherence.

When Sleep Finds You

For those who must wait too long for rest

When the world won't dim,
and the walls hum with other people's nights,
your nerves remain lit—
like a city that forgot
how to turn off its lights.

The suprachiasmatic nucleus,
keeper of circadian time,
searches for signal through static—
craving darkness, craving rhythm,
craving silence that never comes.

Melatonin waits in vain,
held hostage by noise,
by the flicker behind your eyes,
by the cortisol whispering
"Stay alert—this is not safe."

Your brain, once ready to soften,
spins in tight loops of hypervigilance—
neurotransmitters tangled,
norepinephrine pacing the corridors,
acetylcholine too wired for dreams.

Sleep deprivation frays the mind—
a thousand jangled synapses
trying to harmonize without rest.

But still,
when conditions are right—
when the room is quiet,
the air just cool enough,
and trust begins to settle its weight
on your chest like a warm dog,

the descent begins.

A moment comes—
not a decision, but a surrender—
as the thalamus gates the world,
and you fall through your own body
like a stone through deep water.

Slow-wave sleep takes hold,
clearing metabolic waste,
resetting synapses,
rebuilding your emotional scaffolding
beneath the veil of dreaming.

Then comes REM—
your theater of meaning,
your hippocampus humming in rehearsal,
laying down the traces of who you are
and what might come next.

You awaken—eventually—
not healed all at once,
but rewoven,
thread by invisible thread.

Because sleep is not the absence of waking.
It is the brain's most sacred work—
invisible, essential,
a homecoming to the self
that waits in quiet
to be made whole again.

Clinical Postscript

This poem emerged after two sleepless nights in a loud Hamburg hotel. As someone with autism, my sensory system doesn't simply detect sound—it magnifies it. Sudden noises, distant traffic, even hallway movement register as internal alarms. My nervous system, attuned for survival, cannot transition into rest without the signal of safety.

Clinically, this reflects a failure to engage parasympathetic tone. Excess environmental stimulation suppresses melatonin production and keeps cortisol elevated, disrupting the circadian orchestration governed by the suprachiasmatic nucleus. Without this entrainment, even a tired brain remains alert.

Sleep is not a passive default—it's an active neurobiological symphony. During deep NREM sleep, the glymphatic system clears toxins. During REM, the hippocampus organizes memory and emotion. Each phase is a phase of healing, integration, and identity repair.

When sleep does come, especially after deprivation, it isn't just restorative—it's profound. It reaffirms that the world is once again quiet enough to trust.

The Ones Who Cannot Let Down

Some nights,
I lie in the dark like a sentinel,
every nerve strung
as if the walls might betray me.
My body knows the room is safe—
but my nervous system doesn't believe it.

The hum of distant traffic,
a door clicking two rooms down—
it might as well be thunder.
Cortisol coils through my veins,
acetylcholine firing sharp.
The world outside is still,
but inside,
I am galloping.

I think of the horse
who never drops his head—
who scans the horizon
even in the round pen,
ears flicking,
body braced like a bow.
They call him "difficult,"
but I know that stance.

We are the same,
he and I—
unable to let go,
not for lack of sleep or training,
but because the brain

hasn't been convinced
that surrender is safe.

His hippocampus holds
the ghosts of last time,
his amygdala tuned to tones
humans don't hear.
I recognize the look—
not wildness,
but watchfulness.

To ask for softness
in that state
is like asking the tide to rest
while the moon is still pulling.

I, too, have wanted
to fall into sleep like a warm pasture—
to let my limbs forget the day,
to fold into quiet.
But vigilance is a muscle
that doesn't unclench
just because it's tired.

And so I do not command the horse to relax.
I *invite* him
by becoming quiet myself,
by lowering my own breath
so that maybe,
he will feel it.

Peace will come for both of us—
not as a trick,
but as a trust.
A signal that the world

has paused its threats
long enough
for us to come home
to the body.

Clinical Postscript

Hypervigilance—whether in a human lying awake in a hotel or a horse standing alert in a paddock—is not a behavior chosen by will. It is a neurobiological state shaped by experience, threat perception, and nervous system conditioning.

In both species, the amygdala plays a central role in assessing safety. When a past experience, environment, or sensory cue is interpreted as potentially threatening, cortisol and norepinephrine maintain sympathetic arousal, even in the absence of actual danger. The hippocampus, which encodes contextual memory, may reinforce this alert state by recalling moments where safety was breached in similar settings.

For sleep to occur in humans—or for trust to emerge in horses—parasympathetic tone must be dominant. This shift requires cues of safety, not commands. It often depends on co-regulation, where one nervous system, through tone of voice, breath, or body language, can downshift another.

This poem reflects a universal truth for trauma-aware handlers and neurodivergent individuals alike:
relaxation is not a reward for obedience—it is a biological state that must be earned through environment, rhythm, and trust.

Where the Mind Wanders at Night

(on REM sleep and memory consolidation)

You sleep,
but your brain does not.

The hippocampus pulses in waves,
sending its signals forward—
today's moments
looking for a place to belong.

The cortex listens,
rearranges,
threads feeling to fact,
sensation to story.

Theta rhythms rise.
Acetylcholine floods the system.
Eyes flick beneath closed lids,
mapping a world
that never quite was—
and yet feels known.

This is not forgetting.
It is sorting.
Trimming what's no longer needed.
Weaving meaning from fragments.
Making space.

Dreams are not noise.
They are architecture.
Memory,
emotion,
and imagination
in slow rehearsal
for waking life.

Clinical Postscript

REM sleep is a stage of active neurobiological processing. During this phase, the hippocampus and cortex engage in a dialogue, allowing new experiences to be stabilized into long-term memory. This process, known as memory consolidation, helps transform fragmented moments into integrated narrative and meaning.

REM is also crucial for emotional regulation. By reactivating emotionally charged experiences in a neurochemical environment low in norepinephrine, the brain can reprocess those memories with reduced reactivity. Dreams may be a byproduct—or perhaps a reflection—of this activity, representing the brain's effort to sort, link, and sometimes resolve emotional and sensory material.

PGO (ponto-geniculo-occipital) waves, theta rhythms, and acetylcholine surges all mark REM sleep as a distinct and essential time of neuroplastic reorganization. In short, REM isn't escape—it's integration.

The dreaming brain isn't idle.
It is shaping what tomorrow's mind will remember, feel, and understand.

When the Storm Comes Close

—a neuropoem about anxiety

When the storm comes close,
I feel it not in clouds but in current—
Norepinephrine cracks like static in the wires,
edges drawn in sudden spikes—
hyper-alert, eyes wide inside,
scanning for threat where silence dwells.

Cortisol drips like cold rain down my spine,
longer-lasting, slower-burning,
etching dread into my tissues,
engraving urgency into the hours—
even when no teeth, no claws appear.

Glucocorticoid receptors receive the flood,
binding cortisol to quiet the storm—
they're meant to signal: *enough*—
to turn the dial down gently.
But in anxiety, they falter,
and the signal gets lost in the noise.

But beneath the noise,
another frequency murmurs.
Serotonin—
low, steady—
reaches like moss over stone,
trying to smooth the grooves of rumination,
to restore rhythm,
to say: *there is ground beneath you still.*

And if I breathe—
not shallow, not rushed—
but down into the base of me,
the limbic tide begins to slow.

The sympathetic wind, once roaring,
meets a wall of parasympathetic return—
a dampening.
A drawing inward.
A signal whispered through breath:
you are not in danger now.

And in that moment—
though the storm still circles—
I am no longer swept.
I am the place it cannot breach

The Absence

(on the neuroendocrinology of grief)

The body knows
before the mind can bear it—
something is missing.

Not just the hush
where breathing once rose and fell,
or the shared pace
of walks that needed no words.

It is the rupture of rhythm,
the pasture too wide,
the gate unleaned on,
a silence
where morning once began.

Cortisol tides rise and fall—
flattened curves,
stillness under strain.
The nervous system
searches
for a signal
it will never receive.

Yet still—
a dog lingers at the door,
a horse scans the fence line,
a human turns to speak—
then remembers.

Grief is the brain
repeating
what is no longer true,
until it learns
to stop asking.

It burns new grooves
through old routines,
etches silence
into synapse,
and coats every echo
with ache.

And still—
in the hollow that remains,
we listen.
We wait.
We reach
for what mattered.

Clinical Postscript

Grief is a neuroendocrine event as much as an emotional one. Studies have shown that bereavement is associated with elevated cortisol levels, flattened diurnal rhythms, and disrupted morning peaks. These alterations reflect a sustained state of physiological stress, often modulated by how close the bond was with the deceased, the severity of the emotional loss, and individual susceptibility.

Although cortisol is the most studied biomarker, grief undoubtedly affects broader systems. Oxytocin, often linked to attachment and safety, likely plays a role, though empirical research is still emerging. In both humans and non-human animals—horses, dogs, and others—the loss of a bonded partner can lead to behavioral withdrawal, dysregulated affect, and even immune and cardiovascular effects.

This poem captures how the absence of presence leaves a vacuum in shared routines and rhythms. The body, bonded through experience and regulation, is forced to adapt to disconnection. In grief, the nervous system is not just wounded—it is rewiring. The challenge, and the hope, lies in helping that rewiring move toward meaning, resilience, and, eventually, re-connection.

A Still Day Returns

Some moments settle
not in words,
but in the tissues that hold warmth
just a little longer.

Where the air once held a scent—
sunlit hay, skin after rain—
the body still listens.
Not with ears,
but with quiet thresholds
that open when no one is speaking.

Memory is not a photograph.
It's a pattern—
a sequence of signals
preserved in the rhythm of breath,
the way hands soften,
the way the chest yields to calm.

In the presence of safety,
oxytocin flows—
not as romance,
but as recognition.

To walk beside someone
and feel the world slow
is its own kind of neural binding—
limbic circuits learning trust
without instruction.

We do not always know
what we will carry.
But the nervous system remembers
what made us feel whole.

And sometimes,
on a still day,
a breeze will return
with a trace of that feeling—
and the body will answer
as if it had never forgotten.

Clinical Postscript

This poem reflects the neuroscience of implicit memory and somatic recall. Emotional experiences, especially those encoded in safe and attuned relationships, are often stored not as declarative facts but as interoceptive patterns—bodily sensations, shifts in breath, heart rate, and muscle tone. These memories can be reactivated by subtle sensory cues, even in the absence of conscious recollection. Oxytocin, a neuropeptide associated with trust and bonding, plays a key role in this process, reinforcing neural circuits of safety and connection. In this way, the body remembers not the narrative, but the feeling—and sometimes, in stillness, that feeling returns.

All the Signals We Forgot to Follow

The first signal
was not a word—
but warmth.
Skin to skin,
a field of oxytocin blooming
before names
were ever learned.

The second
was gaze—
not to control,
but to tether
our scattered hemispheres
into one
brief unity of presence.

You once trembled
at a sound
you could not name.
The limbic system
does not require language—
only fidelity
to survival.

But you stayed.
You did not run
from the flood.

Instead,
you opened
to the full weight
of your own
interoceptive tide—
each heartbeat
a metronome
for the world
you're still becoming.

Beneath every conscious thought
is a network of whispers—
acetylcholine weaving focus,
serotonin smoothing the storm.

And dopamine—
that ancient light—
illuminates the paths
you did not know
you had the strength
to take.

What remains
isn't memory.
It is pattern,
etched into fascia,
tender in the amygdala,
softened by breath.

You are not
the sum of what happened.
You are the symphony
of what rewired
in response.

So when silence comes,
listen carefully.

That's your brain,
still playing
its secret chords—
rewritten by every kindness
you thought
no one noticed.

Clinical Postscript

This poem explores the silent choreography of brain and body as they navigate emotion, memory, and healing. It follows the neurobiological trail of attachment, attention, and adaptation—where oxytocin, serotonin, dopamine, and acetylcholine become not just chemicals, but currents in the lived music of survival and becoming.

Homecoming Frequencies

I walk the streets where four generations stood—
where porches held voices, and gardens held time.
The soil remembers us,
even when I forget.

Beneath my feet,
the land hums in familiar tones—
not memory,
but recognition.

A frequency of belonging
moves through my being.
My breath deepens.
The sympathetic static quiets,
not through effort,
but through gravity.

The nervous system settles—
not as visitor,
but as native.

It listens to the cadence of wind in the trees,
to light falling across familiar eaves,
to rhythms once woven into cradle songs and farewells.
The lake glimmers nearby—
a mirror of lineage and light.

I do not need to speak.
I only need to stand,
and feel the coherence
of sacred earth received.

This poem was written during a visit to St. Joseph, Michigan, where four generations of my family lived within just four city blocks. The houses, sidewalks, and trees here hold more than passing time—they carry the imprint of lives well lived. Our farms once bordered the town, and the rhythms of work, family, and seasons shaped the legacy that still lingers in this place. Walking these familiar streets, I felt the quiet presence of those who came before me. This poem is both a remembrance and a return—a reflection on continuity, belonging, and the enduring presence of home.

Whiz-Bang Echoes

I turned off the main road
and followed a dirt path
that still knew my name.
It curled like a neural loop
toward the old homestead,
half-forgotten
but encoded deep
in the folds of memory.

There it was—
the farmhouse we once filled
with elbows on tables
and supper prayers.
Now slumped,
its front porch collapsed
like a spine gone brittle,
where Uncle Charlie once sat
in from the fields,
steam rising off coffee
thick as the dusk.

We used to gather there—
cousins claiming creaky chairs,
waiting on supper
served from a kitchen
whose linoleum peeled like sunburn.
Everything came in
shades of brown and white:
a roast, boiled potatoes,
slices of white bread

stacked like blank pages,
whole milk sweating in its jug,
vanilla ice cream melting slowly
beneath Hershey's syrup.
Back then, they said it'd stick to your bones—
now we'd say it sticks to your arteries.

The wash basin waited
like a ritual site—
Lava soap crumbling on the edge,
brush nearby,
braced to scrub
the day's dirt
from knuckles and memory.

Every entrance
sounded the whiz-bang
of the screen door—
a pulse the old house remembered,
each slam a spark
waking it from its quiet,
as voices and footsteps
filled the rooms
and life settled back
into its corners.

That night,
two tribes formed—
those shuffling cards
and laying down dominoes
on the folding table,
and those turned toward
the hum and static
of the hometown Tigers,
black-and-white ghosts

on a flickering TV,
a coat hanger twisting skyward
as antenna.

Uncle Chuck asked
when did players go soft—
"Back in my day,
we kept all five fingers
in the glove."
His voice held
something sacred—
not complaint,
but the tectonic shift
of a world moving on
without asking.

As I drove away,
rearview framing
what the mind could not release,
the neural pathways
lit like fireflies:
a map drawn in
coffee steam,
cracked linoleum,
and the long, slow shimmer
of synapses replaying scenes
that no longer exist, yet never left.

The Horse's Brain and Ours

Let's start with something simple—and profound.
The horse's brain is not a complete mystery.
It is not unknowable.
It is not—despite what some may claim—wild, unpredictable and in need of being dominated, sublimated and over controlled.
The horse is a sensory, emotional, pattern-seeking being.
And in many ways, not so different from us.
When we speak of trust, of fear, of learning, of memory,
communication or connection,
we are not speaking in metaphor.
We are speaking in biology.
Because when we train a horse,
we are not merely shaping behavior.
We are shaping a brain.

A Horse Remembers

She stood alone at the far end of the paddock—still, frozen,
somewhere else.
The same spot she returned to every day.

To most, it looked like a simple habit.
But to me… it was a footprint etched into the nervous system.

You see, a horse doesn't remember the way we do.
There are no words. No timeline. No story.

There is only Sensation. Emotion. Pattern.
And when a moment is flooded with cortisol, fear, and uncertainty,
the memory is etched deep by the amygdala.

Especially after being "*taught a lesson*" more than once.

She wasn't just standing there—
she was checked out, numbed out…
not living in the now,
but trapped in the past.

But there is hope.
With patience, softness, and the right approach—
through safety, consistency, and time—
that memory can be reshaped.

Not erased. Not forgotten.
But softened, reframed, and rewired.

That is the quiet power of working with the brain and nervous system.
Not command, but connection.
Not force, but understanding.
And sometimes, it begins…
by simply standing still.

Perceiving Like a Horse

A horse does not see the world as we do.
Their eyes, set wide on either side,
offer a near-panoramic view—
a living landscape, always in motion.

They do not focus in a tunnel like we do.
They track the broad sweep—
movement along the horizon,
a flicker of light, the ripple of a shadow,
a predator's whisper on the edge of distance.

The horizontal pupil is not just a shape.
It is a strategy.
A tool honed by evolution
to keep the body safe
by watching the world all at once.

In the dark, their world does not disappear.
It softens.
Their retinas, dense with rods,
draw light from the thinnest sliver.
What we call night
is for them a dimly lit room.
They walk it with confidence
while we grope and guess.

Their ears move independently,
sweeping the air like antennae,
searching for frequencies
we no longer hear.

The high-pitched alarm of a fawn,
the wingbeat of an owl—
they register not only the sound,
but its direction, distance, and intent.

Their bodies listen too.
The skin is tuned to subtleties—
a single fly landing,
a breeze shifting from one flank to another.
The tactile neurons beneath their coats
map the world in sensation.
Pressure, warmth, vibration—
each a form of information.

Touch is not simple for a horse.
It is layered.
It can soothe, or startle.
A hand on the withers,
a brush too firm,
a cinch drawn hastily—
these speak volumes
to a nervous system trained for vigilance.

Their lips are fingers.
They explore the earth
not by grabbing, but by grazing,
not by clutching, but by sifting.
A stem of grass, a sprig of yarrow,
a pebble, a thorn—
they sort edible from inedible
with precision that requires no thought,
only the quiet labor of sensation.

Their whiskers—vibrissae—
are not facial ornaments.
They are sensory beacons.
They measure distance, texture,
movement, the contour of objects.
Removing them is like
cutting the fingertips off a blind pianist.

And always, beneath it all,
the hum of arousal—
not stress, not fear—
but readiness.
The locus coeruleus,
the amygdala,
the sympathetic tone—
always assessing,
always poised to act.

This is not weakness.
This is intelligence,
expressed in a language
we rarely understand.

To work with a horse
is to enter this world—
a place of nuance,
of sensing before speaking,
of feeling before doing.

To earn their trust
is to match their awareness
with our own.

And perhaps to remember
that there are other ways
to be intelligent.
Other ways to know the world.

New Trails

The horse was not born knowing the rein,
Nor the feel of a rider, nor yielding to pain.
But the brain—it listens, rewires, adapts,
Forging new pathways from whispers and taps.

Each moment of stillness, each patient release,
Carves out a pattern, a pathway to peace.
The synapse fires, the circuits align,
What was once chaos becomes a design.

A flick of the ear, a softening eye—
Not magic, but neurons giving reply.
Plastic, not fixed, the brain finds its way,
In repetition and rhythm, day after day.

So ride with awareness, shape with intent,
Each cue is a chisel, each breath a lament
Or a hymn—depending on how you train.
You're not just riding the horse. You're riding the brain.

The Dopamine Drift

It begins before the cue—
in the lean of the body,
the flick of an ear,
the moment you both wonder
what might happen next.

Not demand,
but discovery.

The basal ganglia stirs,
tracking the shape of the routine.
Patterns form.
Expectations hum.

And there it is—
a try,
barely more than a shift of weight,
a question asked with the body.

You release.
Timing perfect.
Pressure melts like snow.

And somewhere deep in the midbrain,
dopamine rises—
not in triumph,
but in affirmation.

Yes.
This is the path.
This is the way.

The horse blinks,
chews,
lowers their head.
Not in submission,
but in the arc of pendulation.

Learning,
true learning,
feels like this—
not forced,
but followed.
Not driven,
but drawn.

Step by step,
loop by loop,
you build a habit not of obedience
but of seeking.

And in that seeking
lies the quiet joy
of a nervous system
allowed to explore,
to choose,
to change.

This is the drift—
the neurochemical current
that shapes behavior
without breaking spirit.

And it flows both ways.

In Step

There is a rhythm in the horse
that isn't taught,
only felt—
in the sway of a walk,
the lift of a trot,
the quiet of a shared breath.

The horse does not seek to lead or follow—
only to *be* in time,
to move with what is true
and feel the weight of presence balanced,
light as a whisper on the back.

When we carry ourselves with balance,
they adjust their own.
When our signals are quiet and consistent,
they soften and listen.
Their bodies respond in moments—
to breath, to posture,
to the space we give or take.

They're always seeking rhythm,
even when we disrupt it.
Always willing
to return to center
if we'll meet them there.

But when we rush, or freeze, or grasp too tight—
when our minds wander or our hands demand—
the rhythm falters.
The dance is lost.

Yet still,
the horse waits.
Soft-eyed, listening,
ready to begin again.
Willing to meet us
where movement becomes music,
and silence,
a shared note of understanding.

The Dance Between Loops

There is no telepathy here—
no mind-reading,
no whispered thought leaping
from my skull to his.

When my calf shifts,
his flank yields.
When I breathe deeper,
his spine softens.

Beneath flesh and fur,
the basal ganglia hum—
his and mine—
quiet engines of practiced motion,
patterns emerging
as neurons fire in tandem,
each network reshaping,
reflecting the rhythm of the other.

Without thought,
the signal flows—
cortex to calf,
flank to forebrain.
Sensation shapes connection,
and each shared rhythm
deepens the groove.
Neurons that fire together
begin to wire as one.

Impulses become words.
Synapses, punctuation.
Connection reshapes us both
in the shared language of neurochemistry.

In time, our loops entwine:
two sensory-motor systems
learning the same rhythm,
mirroring reflex with response,
anticipation with adaptation.

There are moments—
as thought dissolves into rhythm,
and our circuits align—
that I forget
where I end
and he begins.

Regulators

(for horses and humans seeking balance)

I. Baseline

A flank twitches.
The morning holds its breath.
The horse, still drowsy from sleep,
shifts weight—left hind, right front—
without urgency.
No command, no cue.
Just the nervous system listening
to the temperature of the world
and adjusting, quietly.

In your own body,
you sip from stillness—
a pulse, a breath,
glucose whispering across a membrane.
Not striving.
Just staying.
The miracle is not in the action—
but in the return.

II. Forecast

But the wind shifts.
And so does the body.
A rustle in the brush becomes a signal.
Cortisol walks in,
not to frighten,
but to prepare.
Heart rate picks up,
muscle tone holds.

The horse isn't panicked—
just *ready*.

You feel it too—
a sudden email,
a sound too loud,
a thought too sharp.
Prediction engines spool inside your skull.
You adjust,
tighten,
prime.
Not because you're afraid—
but because you've survived.

III. Recovery

Later—
when the noise passes,
and the pasture softens,
the horse returns to grazing.
Lips moving over grass
as if nothing happened.
But something did.
The body practiced returning.

You too can return—
if breath is offered space,
if you let the exhale
linger.
Not as performance.
But as recalibration.
Homeostasis is not perfection.
It is forgiveness,
repeated.

IV. Shared System
Horse and human.
Different species.
Same strategies.
Fluid regulators
in a changing world.
The work is not in staying calm.
The work is in returning
without judgment.

And in this—
you are not alone.
The horse,
beside you,
is doing the same.

Clinical Postscript

This poem explores the neurobiological processes of homeostasis, allostasis, and self-regulation as shared mechanisms in horses and humans. It invites the reader to recognize regulation not as a fixed state, but as a dynamic process of physiological and neural adjustment.

Read with attention to your own interoceptive cues—breath, muscle tone, and emotional valence—as you move through each section. The horse's nervous system, like ours, does not seek constancy, but adaptive flexibility.

Regulation is not the absence of disturbance—it is the capacity to recalibrate.

Islands of Doubt

I lost my form
trying to conform
to schemas that stifled signal—
top-down models
that drowned the raw data
of my lived experience.

I wore composure
like an overlay—
prefrontal varnish
on limbic unrest—
until the system reached overload
and peripheral cues lit up
like hazard lights in the dark.

There used to be clarity—
a clean split
between sensation and story,
but the brain doesn't work that way.
It predicts.
It hallucinates.
It calls guesses "truth"
until the guess no longer fits.

Facts don't arrive all at once.
They drip—
like neurotransmitters across a cleft,
like revelations in REM.
They twist through memory,
reshape what once felt certain.

I built myself
on control loops—
feedforward illusions
of mastery.
But now I am
an island of uncertainty—
adrift and alert,
bitter medicine dissolving
on the tongue of awareness.

Still I pause.
Still I listen—
not for rescue,
but for neural repair.

Because when the signal returns
through closed eyes and open systems,
I will not reach
for certainty as shield or sword.

I will become the waveform—
the embodied hypothesis,
further evolving with ambiguity,
rewired by what I am now willing to feel

if only we listen,
and feel,
and stay.

Clinical Postscript

The brain is not a passive receiver of reality—it is an active constructor. Every moment is a best guess, built from prior experience and shaped by the body's current state. What we call "truth" is often a prediction that hasn't yet been contradicted.

In times of emotional dissonance, when signals no longer match expectations, we may experience this as anxiety, disorientation, or doubt. But doubt is not a defect—it is a neurobiological opening. A rupture in certainty that allows for reconstruction.

This poem traces the journey through that rupture: from the collapse of control to the emergence of further evolution. From top-down imposition to bottom-up integration. From fear of the unknown to curiosity about what might rewire us—

The Moment Before the Map

There is a hush
before a thought becomes a shape,
before the signal chooses its path.

A neuron waits—
not in silence, but in readiness,
its dendrites listening like branches in wind
for a reason to bloom.

This is not memory.
Not yet.
This is the field before the footstep,
the breath before the word.

Perception arrives
not as truth,
but as a truce
between body and brain—
a temporary treaty
signed in the ink of experience.

You call it now,
but it is always becoming—
a synaptic sketch
of what might be real.

And if you pause
long enough
to feel the space between firings,
you will find
that awareness is not the spark—
but the gap.

That is where the map begins.

Clinical Postscript

This piece explores the pre-conscious space where perception forms and neural representations emerge.

Threshold Frequency

For those who follow the scientist who dared to feel

I brought credentials to the gate—
a name etched in data,
a mind trained to measure
what could be proven,
published,
peer-reviewed.

But I began to hear
something unspeakable
in the silence between synapses.
Not a fact—
but a frequency.

Not a proof—
but a pulse
that said:
step closer.

At first, I resisted.
Called it noise.
Then metaphor.
Then madness.

But the current did not need belief.
It only needed my openness.

So I crossed.
With my science intact.
Not abandoned—
but amplified.

And here,
in this new field,
I found others listening, too.

Not to me—
but *through me.*

This is where the books begin.
This is where the method dissolves
into meaning.

This is where we stop
studying the brain—
and begin
becoming it.

Transmitter

—a neuropoem about stillness, signal, and the unseen current

I sit right down.
Not in boredom,
not in prayer,
but in that humming place
where thought hasn't yet been born.

The river moves without my asking—
not water, but current—
an unseen stream of signal
moving through the roots of things.

I wait for it.
Not with fingers poised to strike,
but with ears
tuned to frequencies
most don't believe in.

The gift arrives
not in sound or vision,
but in coherence—
a trembling alignment
between self and source.

And when it does,
I have to decide:
will I open my mouth
and let it speak through me—
risking that what I say
might ripple too deep,

dislodge foundations,
turn the lights on too fast?

Sometimes, I stay quiet
out of mercy.
Not everyone is ready
to feel the shape
of what I've felt.

But still I tune,
still I anchor,
still I wait in the quiet
like a stamen in bloom,
knowing that some breeze
will come
to carry this pollen
to the next
fertile
mind.

The Illusion of the Same

You are not the same
as the signal that passed through you yesterday.
That chain of voltage,
those fleeting ions,
have long rerouted,
leaving behind new potentials
in their wake.

Your brain—
a command center sealed in shadow—
has never seen the world.
It lives in silence,
bathed in cerebrospinal tides,
surrounded by bone and dura,
utterly dependent
on what the senses deliver.

You do not perceive reality.
You construct it.
Sensory organs transduce energy—
light into voltage,
vibration into frequency,
pressure into chemical release.
These signals are routed
through ascending pathways,
shaped by filters of attention, memory,
and internal state.
What reaches awareness
is not the world itself,
but the brain's best guess.

Experience doesn't just live in memory.
It becomes structure.
Trauma alters thresholds.
Joy opens gates.
Serotonin sets the emotional tone.
Dopamine points to reward.
Oxytocin marks a moment as safe.

And so, the brain rewires.
With every action,
with every pattern repeated or broken,
it shapes itself—
myelin thickens,
synapses strengthen or dissolve.
You become your own experiment
in adaptation.

The myth is that you are constant—
a stable identity riding the waves.
But you are the waves:
a moving field of signals,
an unfolding map
drawn in real time.

To grow is to guide the current.
To notice beauty,
to dwell in peace,
is to amplify the very signals
that sculpt the nervous system anew.

You are not who you were.
You are not who you will be.
But with intention,

you can become
someone your future self
will thank you for.

The Gravity of Signal

When I yield to the pull of the Universe,
I do not seek calm.
I remember it.
I return to it.
I become it.

A greater current carries me.
External noise dissolves,
falling away beneath
the weight of coherence.

What once echoed
through limbic halls—
anxious footfalls,
forgotten alarms—
is now only residue.

Recognized.
Observed.
Released.

I do not wrestle shadows.
I do not argue with echoes.
I return to signal—
to frequency and stillness.

My nervous system becomes a tuning fork
for truth.
I am not the noise.
I am the note.

Altitude Reset

Argument, accusation—
a storm inside the skull.
Blame flares,
voices rise,
nervous system spikes into red alert.
Too much sound,
too many signals.
The brain locks its doors.

So Kip and I go—
out.
Up.

Each switchback peels a layer.
Noise thins.
Breath drops anchor,
deeper with the climb,
slower, wiser.
Nature lends her rhythm
to a system seeking homeostasis.

We find a boulder
—midway between earth and sky—
and sit.

The trees don't react.
The clouds don't defend.
Nothing explains itself.

Perspective expands
like the landscape below.
My mind, once crowded,
now mirrors the open sky.

I get almost sleepy
in the stillness,
until the smallest of rainclouds
kisses my skin.
Even that feels like medicine.

Descending,
I notice wildflowers
I must have walked past.
Were they always there?
Or has awareness returned
with the clearing of internal fog?

By the time we reach the bottom,
the fight feels distant,
a flicker in a system
now reset.
What mattered up close
dissolves in the view
from a higher place.

Kip's Trail Lessons: "The High View"

We made the climb today—
me and Kip—
up the ridge where stone and silence meet,
where the wind moves steady through the pines,
and the air, crisp and clean,
carries a bite sharp enough to bring tears to the eyes—
not sadness, just clarity.

Kip ranged ahead as always,
nimble as ever despite her years—
still moving like a mountain sheep,
sure-footed, fluid,
pausing every so often
to glance back,
waiting for me to catch up.

She seemed brighter up there,
more alive—
energized by the open world around us,
her senses fully engaged:
nose to the breeze,
ears flicking at distant calls,
eyes sweeping the mountainside with calm precision.

And when we reached the top—
eight thousand feet above the canyon floor—
we turned to look.

The ranch lay below us,
fenced pastures shaped by stewardship,
laid out with the kind of thought that listens to the land.
The horses grazed in stillness,
each a quiet presence folded into the earth's rhythm.

Pines and junipers stood sentinel at our backs,
their scent rising pungent in the breeze.
A red-tailed hawk rode the thermals overhead—
not hunting, not rushing—
just part of the sky,
her gaze steady,
as if the wind itself turned in deference to her flight.

Kip stood beside me then,
breathing in what I was breathing in:
the vastness,
the stillness,
the shared belonging.

This is the kind of moment that restores the brain,
not by effort,
but by remembering what it evolved to do—
to listen,
to perceive,
to dwell in the real.

And this is not rare for me.
This is the practice—
to hike, to feel, to witness.
To let the mind stretch out
like Kip does when we get home—
content,
fulfilled,
and tuned once more to what matters.

Brain, Not Bronc

"We're not breaking colts—we're building them.
We're not shaping behavior—we're shaping the brain.
We shape the environment so the horse finds its own relief.
We shape the try.

This is brain, not bronc."

You Are the Ongoing Pattern

There is no final form.
Only unfolding.

Your brain is not a record.
It is a rhythm.
A question
answered
by how you live.

What you attend to,
you become.

What you feel,
you shape.

Keep going.
The pattern is still forming.

GLOSSARY OF NEURAL TERMS

A guide to terms used in the poems and postscripts of this book.
Written for clarity and grounded understanding.

Acetylcholine
A neurotransmitter involved in attention, learning, and voluntary muscle movement. It enhances focus and supports the brain's readiness for task engagement.

Amygdala
A small, almond-shaped brain structure involved in detecting threats, processing fear, and assigning emotional relevance to stimuli.

Axon
The long projection of a neuron that transmits electrical impulses away from the cell body to other neurons, muscles, or glands.

Basal Ganglia
A group of deep brain nuclei involved in movement control, procedural learning, and habit formation.

Brainstem
The most evolutionarily ancient part of the brain, responsible for autonomic functions such as breathing, heart rate, and arousal.

Cerebellum
A brain structure at the back of the head that coordinates movement, balance, and motor learning.

Cingulate Gyrus
Part of the limbic system involved in emotion processing, pain perception, and behavioral regulation.

Cortisol
A steroid hormone released by the adrenal glands in response to stress. It mobilizes energy but can impair regulation if chronically elevated.

Dendrite
The branch-like extension of a neuron that receives signals from other neurons at synapses.

Dopamine
A neurotransmitter involved in reward, motivation, movement, and learning. It helps drive goal-directed behavior and pattern recognition.

Glia (Glial Cells)
Non-neuronal cells that support, nourish, insulate, and protect neurons. They play essential roles in homeostasis, immune defense, and neural repair.

Hippocampus
A curved structure in the medial temporal lobe important for forming new memories and processing spatial information.

Homeostasis
The body's internal regulation system that maintains physiological balance across systems like temperature, hydration, and pH.

Hypothalamus
A small brain region that regulates hormones, appetite, body temperature, and the autonomic nervous system.

Insula
A brain region involved in interoception—the ability to sense internal bodily states—as well as emotion and empathy.

Limbic System
A network of brain structures involved in emotion, memory, and behavior. Includes the amygdala, hippocampus, and parts of the cingulate cortex.

Mirror Neurons
Neurons that fire both when performing an action and when observing the same action performed by others. They are associated with imitation, empathy, and social learning.

Neuroplasticity
The brain's ability to adapt and change by forming new neural connections in response to experience, learning, or injury.

Norepinephrine
A neurotransmitter and hormone that increases alertness, attention, and readiness to act. It is involved in the body's fight-or-flight response.

Parasympathetic Nervous System
The branch of the autonomic nervous system responsible for relaxation, digestion, and recovery following stress.

Pituitary Gland
The brain's "master gland," it regulates hormone production throughout the body and is influenced by signals from the hypothalamus.

Prefrontal Cortex
The front part of the brain responsible for executive functions like decision-making, attention, planning, empathy, and impulse control.

REM Sleep (Rapid Eye Movement Sleep)
A sleep stage associated with vivid dreaming, brain activity, and memory consolidation. It plays a critical role in emotional processing.

Serotonin
A neurotransmitter involved in mood regulation, emotional stability, sleep, and overall well-being.

Suprachiasmatic Nucleus (SCN)
A cluster of neurons in the hypothalamus that controls circadian rhythms by responding to light and regulating the sleep-wake cycle.

Sympathetic Nervous System
The branch of the autonomic nervous system that prepares the body for action in response to perceived threat. Activates heart rate, respiration, and energy mobilization.

Synapse
The gap between neurons where communication occurs via neurotransmitter release and receptor binding.

Vagus Nerve
The longest cranial nerve, central to the parasympathetic nervous system. It helps regulate heart rate, digestion, and emotional calming.

Printed in Dunstable, United Kingdom

71350570R00068